GET IN TOUCH

Bring the *Armed With Gratefulness* Gratitude workshop to your area

tcmason@imabeautifulweirdo.com

Follow on Social Media

Facebook: imabeautifulweirdo
Instagram: @imabeautifulweirdo
#beautifulweirdo #immaG

Created by T.C Mason
Published by Beautiful Weirdo
ISBN 978-0-9976572-5-8
Copyright© 2019 Beautiful Weirdo

Discover other books by T.C. Mason of Beautiful Weirdo

The Making of Beautiful Weirdo: Nuggets to Push Thru Life And Make the Awkward Beautiful

bit.ly/makingofabeautifulweirdo
www.shopbeautifulweirdo.com

Beautiful Weirdo
www.imabeautifulweirdo.com

DEDICATION

Grateful for life's lessons that led to this destination and for my framily who've always been my cheerleaders encouraging me along the way. Special thanks to my husband, who is my best friend and is a constant entry amongst my grateful posts.

"ENJOY THE LITTLE THINGS, FOR ONE DAY YOU MAY LOOK BACK AND REALIZE THEY WERE THE BIG THINGS."

-Rober Brault

TABLE OF CONTENTS

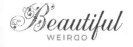

5 REASONS

You'll Love The Armed
With Gratefulness Journal

1. QUICK & EASY:

Takes less than 5 minutes to acknowledge and write down your thoughts. There's no long drawn out plan that requires you to purchase a whole bunch of accessories, etc. You can get started right now, in the next second or minute!

2. YOU'RE IN CONTROL:

You decide what to acknowledge. No one controls your gratefulness, but you. Somedays it you may be long-winded and "deep," and other times it may be as simple as finding a pen that worked when you needed it. Big or small, this is your life and it's up to you.

3. GATEWAY TO POSITIVE EMOTIONS:

Studies have shown, that gratefulness is the gateway that leads to the experience of other emotions. More specifically, over the past two decades researchers have connected gratefulness to an increase in overall well-being and connectedness (Emmons & McCullough, 2003), increase in motivation to help others (Grant & Gino, 2010), increase in subjective well-being, positive outlook on life and decrease in materialism (Lambert, et al., 2009), better psychological functioning and well-being (Rosmarin, Pirutinksy, Cohen, Galler, & Krumei, 2011), being happier, having better moods, and positive affect (Watkins, Woodard, Stone, & Kolts, 2003), reduced stress (Liao, 2018), filling positive emotional voids

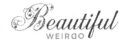

and reduction in depressive symptoms (Lambert, Fincham, & Stillman, 2012; McCollough, Emmons, & Tsang, 2002). All of this from being grateful? Yes, what a powerful weapon. Wow!

4. INCREASE YOUR SELF-ESTEEM:

When you successfully complete a task, it builds confidence and momentum for the next thing. Our brains are so awesome that it says, well if I can do this...then I can also do that!

5. YOU'LL IMPROVE & CHANGE YOUR BRAIN FOR THE BETTER

Your brain is a computer and it loves to connect patterns, routines, and make associations. With that being said, you can train your brain to think more positively. When you consistently do the gratefulness exercises, you will find that your brain will automatically search for the good in every situation.

As a clinical mental health therapist, I have always been intrigued with how people cope with changes, challenges, stress, and traumas in their life. It seemed some people would have challenging situations and get through them fairly well, whereas others would become devastated and depressed and were unable to move forward with their lives. It was like they were trapped, and it was hard witnessing people suffer from depression as it can affect so many domains in life including feelings, thinking, and the ability to handle routine activities of everyday life, such as sleeping, eating, or working (National Institute of Health, 2018; Southwick, Vythilingam, & Charney, 2005; World Health Organization, 2018). Yet, depression affects more than 300 hundred billion people globally, and this number is steadily growing (World Health Organization, 2018). Out of all the people it affects, it affects more women than men as it occurs twice as often in women than in men (Murray & Lopez, 1996; World Health Organization, n.d.). After seeing the detrimental effects of depression at my private practice, I began the quest to be an active part of the solution to help develop and provide solutions and interventions to reduce stressors and symptoms of depression.

One of the things I noticed when counseling individuals who were overwhelmed with stress and or exhibiting symptoms of depression, is how the simple practice of being grateful and including things that brought them joy, decreased their depressive symptoms, increased positive emotions, and allowed them to shift

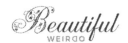

perspectives and see things differently. In contrast, I noticed that when clients did not include the things that brought them joy or did not reflect on the things that were going well in everyday life, they seemed to be more stressed. So, it got me thinking, if gratefulness can increase positive feelings and change perspectives for the better, how come we aren't using this intervention more often? Thus, began my curiosity and journey to learn, develop, and implement tools to empower people thru the usage of positive psychology, with gratefulness being one of them.

I'm currently a student studying to obtain a doctorate in general psychology. More specifically, I am interested in educating diverse populations (i.e. especially women) on the power of happiness, positive emotions, and positive psychology interventions. I am seeking to become a leading scholar-practitioner who develops programming, research, and interventions that demonstrate the effectiveness of using happiness and positive psychology as a buffer and a coping mechanism to lessen the effects of stress and symptoms of depression. So, as I learn effective tools and interventions, I will share them with the world. I take this war on stress related disorders seriously and it's time that we increase awareness on the tools to combat this worldwide phenomenon.

T.C Mason, LICSW, LCSW-C
Health & Happiness Strategist

Date

Write the date. It helps to track patterns & helps you to stay on track. When you can see your consistency, it creates a momentum. Also, your brain loves routines.

Affirmation

Sets the target for the day. The goal is to prime your brain with a positive statement, so you can aim to reach it. Your brain likes to achieve goals, so give it direction. Also, when you prime your brain for the day with positivity it starts your day off on the right track and sets the course for the day.

Writing

Writing helps you to remember and be more honest with your feelings. Your brain has the habit of holding on to intense feelings and so it is easier to recall negative things (the brain is trying to remember the things that cause you harm, so it can protect you). When you write, you are engaging in a process to remind yourself of all the positive things that were covered by your brain's attempt to protect you.

4 Things You're Grateful 4

Sets the ball in motion so you can reflect on gratefulness. Jot down at least 4....but you can add more. You'll find that one thought of gratefulness may lead to another or another positive emotion. As you engage in gratitude, you will become more optimistic about life.

"Yeah, I did that"

Reflection from the day before about something that went well. It's important to learn how to be your own cheerleader. Training your brain to acknowledge something positive about you every day, also trains your brain to actively look for something positive about you every day. Also, a major characteristic of depression is all or nothing thinking, so in acknowledging, "yeah, I did that," you are training your brain to see the positive in yourself and in all situations.

Ready. Aim. Write.

#immaG

GRATITUDE RESULTS IN

Better sleep

Improved relationships

Better physical health

Better subjective well-being

Better psychological functioning

Less physical symptoms or ailments

Increase in positive emotions

Happier life

Decrease in negative emotions

Ready. Aim. Write.

#immaG

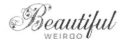

GRATEFUL PEOPLE ARE

Higher in positive emotions and life satisfaction

Lower in negative emotions such as depression, anxiety, and envy

More empathic, forgiving, helpful, and supportive

Less focused on the pursuit of materialistic goals

More spiritually and religiously minded

Consistently more extraverted, more agreeable, and less neurotic than that of their less grateful counterparts

(McCollough, Emmons, & Tsang, 2002)

Ready. Aim. Write.

#immaG

"NO MATTER WHAT
THE SITUATION IS...
CLOSE YOUR EYES
AND THINK OF ALL
OF THE THINGS IN
YOUR LIFE YOU
COULD BE GRATEFUL
FOR RIGHT NOW."

-Deepak Chopra

I'm optimistic & I face my days with a smile.

○ _____

○ _____

○ _____

○ _____

YEAH! I DID THAT!

I feel the fear & do what I need to do anyway because I'm brave. #scareddoitanyway

○ _____

○ _____

○ _____

○ _____

YEAH! I DID THAT!

DATE

There is no one like me & so, my existence is important & needed here on this earth.

WHAT ARE YOU GRATEFUL FOR TODAY?

○ _____
○ _____
○ _____
○ _____

YEAH! I DID THAT!

DATE

I'm the sun & I carry rays of light wherever I go.

WHAT ARE YOU GRATEFUL FOR TODAY?

○ _____
○ _____
○ _____
○ _____

YEAH! I DID THAT!

I'm a fighter & I kick at the darkness until it bleeds daylight.

○ _____

○ _____

○ _____

○ _____

YEAH! I DID THAT!

WHAT ARE YOU GRATEFUL FOR TODAY?

I'm assertive in advocating for myself & speaking my truth.

○ _____

○ _____

○ _____

○ _____

YEAH! I DID THAT!

WHAT ARE YOU GRATEFUL FOR TODAY?

"GRATITUDE... CAN TURN A MEAL INTO A FEAST, A HOUSE INTO A HOME, A STRANGER INTO A FRIEND."

-Melody Beattie

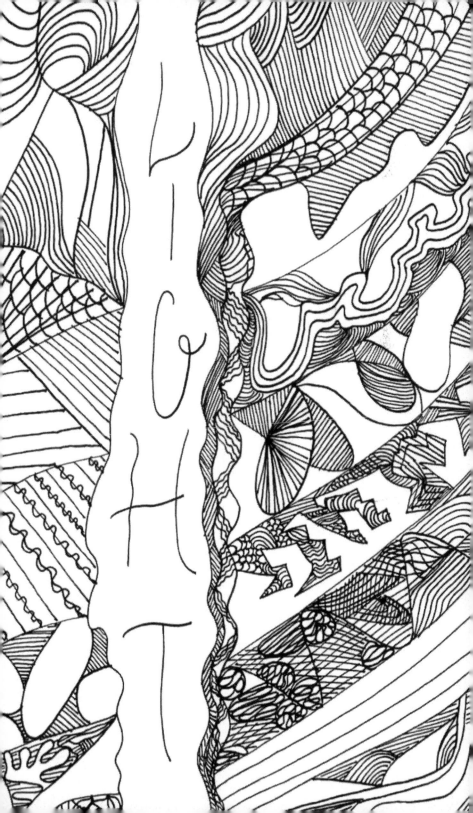

I'm courageous in who I'm becoming.

WHAT ARE YOU GRATEFUL FOR TODAY?

- ◯ _____
- ◯ _____
- ◯ _____
- ◯ _____

YEAH! I DID THAT!

I'm forgiving & I allow hurt to grow me...not stop me.

WHAT ARE YOU GRATEFUL FOR TODAY?

- ◯ _____
- ◯ _____
- ◯ _____
- ◯ _____

YEAH! I DID THAT!

I'm strategic & make the necessary sacrifices to be great.

- ◯ _____
- ◯ _____
- ◯ _____
- ◯ _____

YEAH! I DID THAT!

I'm confident in the God I serve & I trust Him.

- ◯ _____
- ◯ _____
- ◯ _____
- ◯ _____

YEAH! I DID THAT!

"GRATITUDE IS AN ANTIDOTE TO NEGATIVE EMOTIONS, A NEUTRALIZER OF ENVY, HOSTILITY, WORRY AND IRRITATION. IT IS SAVORING; IT IS NOT TAKING THINGS FOR GRANTED; IT IS PRESENT ORIENTED."

-Sonja Lyubomirsky

DID YOU KNOW...

Gratitude leads to better sleep.

"When falling asleep, grateful people are less likely to think negative and worrying thoughts, and more likely to think positive thoughts (Wood, Joseph, Lloyd, & Atkins, 2009, p. 46)."

Ready. Aim. Write.

#immaG

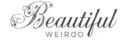

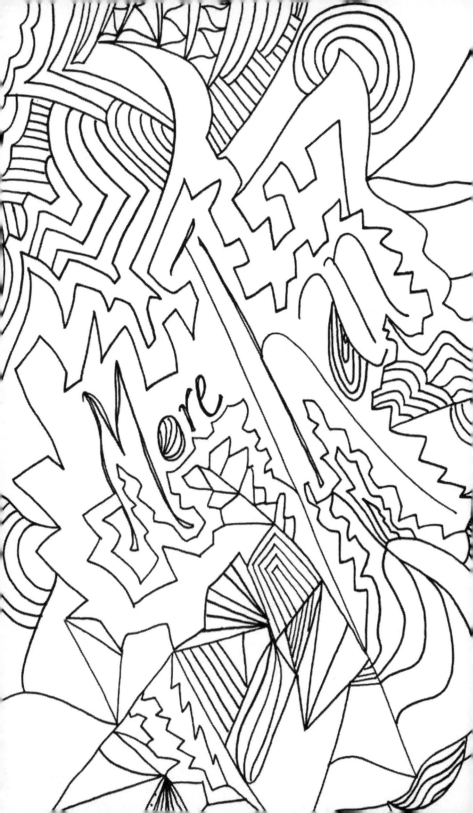

"GRATITUDE FOR
THE PRESENT
MOMENT AND THE
FULLNESS OF LIFE

NOW IS TRUE

PROSPERITY."

-Eckhart Tolle

DATE

I'm consistent & keep pressing, knowing good results will come.

WHAT ARE YOU GRATEFUL FOR TODAY?

○ _____

○ _____

○ _____

○ _____

YEAH! I DID THAT!

DATE

I'm wonderfully made & God has engineered me to soar & excel in life.

WHAT ARE YOU GRATEFUL FOR TODAY?

○ _____

○ _____

○ _____

○ _____

YEAH! I DID THAT!

I'm flexible with my creativity;
I can color in & outside the lines.

○ _____

○ _____

○ _____

○ _____

YEAH! I DID THAT!

WHAT ARE YOU GRATEFUL FOR TODAY?

I'm intentional & I surround myself with
people who love & encourage me.

○ _____

○ _____

○ _____

○ _____

YEAH! I DID THAT!

WHAT ARE YOU GRATEFUL FOR TODAY?

"THE MOST POWERFUL WEAPON AGAINST DAILY BATTLES IS FINDING THE COURAGE TO BE GRATEFUL ANYWAY."

Unknown

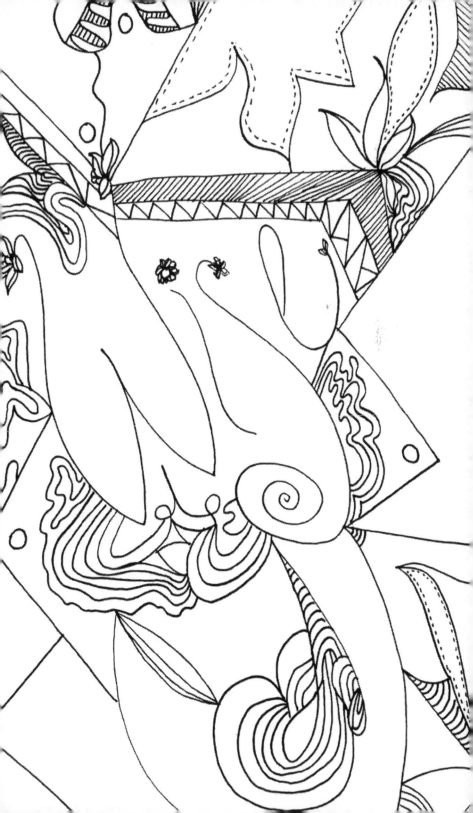

DATE

I'm living & life happens through me.

WHAT ARE YOU GRATEFUL FOR TODAY?

- ◯ _____
- ◯ _____
- ◯ _____
- ◯ _____

YEAH! I DID THAT!

DATE

I'm ambitious & go after opportunities.

WHAT ARE YOU GRATEFUL FOR TODAY?

- ◯ _____
- ◯ _____
- ◯ _____
- ◯ _____

YEAH! I DID THAT!

I'm grateful & my spirit leads to success.

○ _____
○ _____
○ _____
○ _____

YEAH! I DID THAT!

WHAT ARE YOU GRATEFUL FOR TODAY?

I'm a daily examiner of my spirit.

○ _____
○ _____
○ _____
○ _____

YEAH! I DID THAT!

WHAT ARE YOU GRATEFUL FOR TODAY?

"I AM GRATEFUL FOR WHAT I AM AND HAVE. MY THANKSGIVING IS PERPETUAL."

-Henry David Thoreau

DID YOU KNOW...

Gratitude improves relationships.

Expressing gratitude is positively linked
to relationship satisfaction.

Ready. Aim. Write.

#immaG

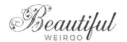

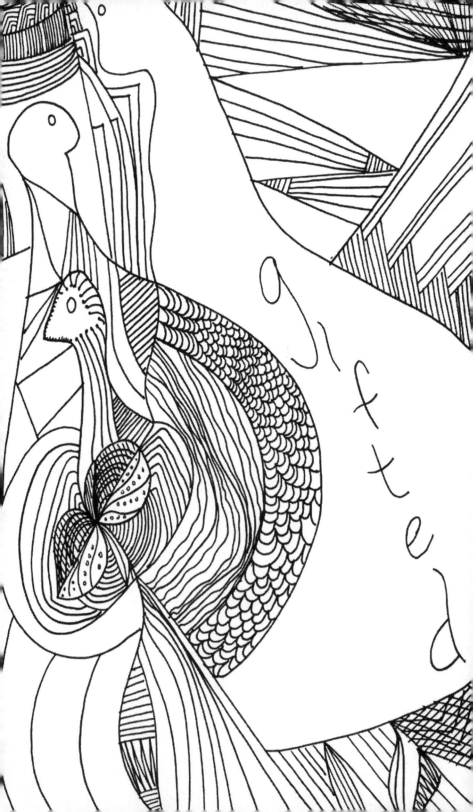

"YOU SIMPLY WILL NOT BE THE SAME PERSON TWO MONTHS FROM NOW AFTER CONSCIOUSLY GIVING THANKS EACH DAY FOR THE ABUNDANCE THAT EXISTS IN YOUR LIFE. AND YOU WILL HAVE SET IN MOTION AN ANCIENT SPIRITUAL LAW: THE MORE YOU HAVE AND ARE GRATEFUL FOR, THE MORE WILL BE GIVEN YOU."

-Sarah Ban Breathnach

I'm honest with myself & I express myself honestly.

WHAT ARE YOU GRATEFUL FOR TODAY?

- ◯ _____
- ◯ _____
- ◯ _____
- ◯ _____

YEAH! I DID THAT!

I'm giving with a mindset of abundance.

WHAT ARE YOU GRATEFUL FOR TODAY?

- ◯ _____
- ◯ _____
- ◯ _____
- ◯ _____

YEAH! I DID THAT!

I'm trusting & I let go the need to control the outcome.

○ _____

○ _____

○ _____

○ _____

YEAH! I DID THAT!

WHAT ARE YOU GRATEFUL FOR TODAY?

I'm free & other's opinions don't hold me hostage.

○ _____

○ _____

○ _____

○ _____

YEAH! I DID THAT!

WHAT ARE YOU GRATEFUL FOR TODAY?

"GRATITUDE IS ONE OF THE MOST POWERFUL HUMAN EMOTIONS. ONCE EXPRESSED, IT CHANGES ATTITUDE, BRIGHTENS OUTLOOK, AND BROADENS OUR PERSPECTIVE."

-Germany Kent

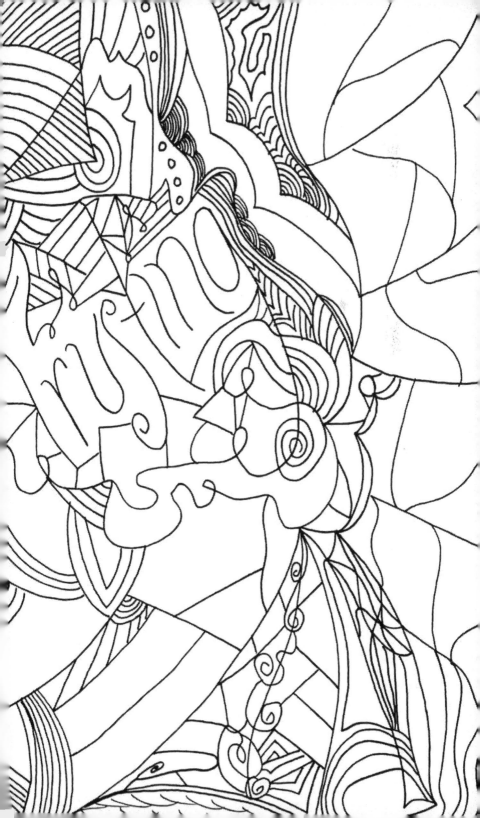

I'm moving forward in every area of my life.

WHAT ARE YOU GRATEFUL FOR TODAY?

- ◯ _____
- ◯ _____
- ◯ _____
- ◯ _____

YEAH! I DID THAT!

I'm a breaker of generational curses.

WHAT ARE YOU GRATEFUL FOR TODAY?

- ◯ _____
- ◯ _____
- ◯ _____
- ◯ _____

YEAH! I DID THAT!

I'm fearless and ask for yes in the face of no.

○ _____

○ _____

○ _____

○ _____

YEAH! I DID THAT!

I'm a protector of my joy as it is my strength.

○ _____

○ _____

○ _____

○ _____

YEAH! I DID THAT!

"IT'S NOT POSSIBLE
TO EXPERIENCE
CONSTANT
EUPHORIA, BUT IF
YOU'RE GRATEFUL,
YOU CAN FIND
HAPPINESS IN
EVERYTHING."

-Pharrell Williams

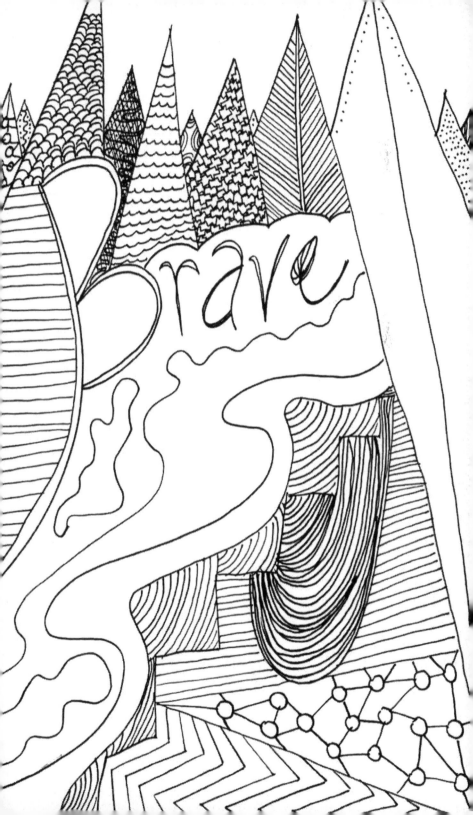

I'm amazing & God is tickled at the thought of me.

WHAT ARE YOU GRATEFUL FOR TODAY?

- ◯ _____
- ◯ _____
- ◯ _____
- ◯ _____

YEAH! I DID THAT!

I'm a mathematician adding greatness to my life & subtracting foolishness from my life.

WHAT ARE YOU GRATEFUL FOR TODAY?

- ◯ _____
- ◯ _____
- ◯ _____
- ◯ _____

YEAH! I DID THAT!

I'm content in stillness, it is my quiet power.

○ _____
○ _____
○ _____
○ _____

YEAH! I DID THAT!

WHAT ARE YOU GRATEFUL FOR TODAY?

I'm a seeker of opportunities to laugh because laughter is my medicine.

○ _____
○ _____
○ _____
○ _____

YEAH! I DID THAT!

WHAT ARE YOU GRATEFUL FOR TODAY?

"GRATITUDE IS THE HEALTHIEST OF ALL HUMAN EMOTIONS. THE MORE YOU EXPRESS GRATITUDE FOR WHAT YOU HAVE, THE MORE LIKELY YOU WILL HAVE EVEN MORE TO EXPRESS GRATITUDE FOR."

-Zig Ziglar

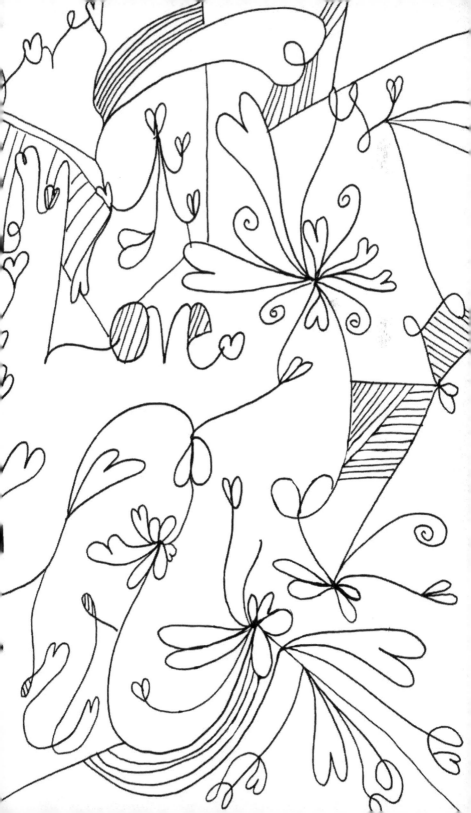

I'm gracious with myself and time.

WHAT ARE YOU GRATEFUL FOR TODAY?

○ _____
○ _____
○ _____
○ _____

YEAH! I DID THAT!

I honor each minute & allow it to be & don't stuff it to capacity.

WHAT ARE YOU GRATEFUL FOR TODAY?

○ _____
○ _____
○ _____
○ _____

YEAH! I DID THAT!

I'm pushing past the old me to uncover the real me.

○ _____

○ _____

○ _____

○ _____

YEAH! I DID THAT!

WHAT ARE YOU GRATEFUL FOR TODAY?

I'm open & receptive to new ideas & new ways of thinking.

○ _____

○ _____

○ _____

○ _____

YEAH! I DID THAT!

WHAT ARE YOU GRATEFUL FOR TODAY?

"GRATEFULNESS IS THE MAGNIFYING GLASS TO HELP YOU SEE AND APPRECIATE LIFE."

-T.C. Mason

DID YOU KNOW...

Gratitude reduces depressive symptoms

Gratitude decreases reports of depressive symptoms by prompting people to reframe otherwise negative experiences as potentially positive experiences. This reframing, in turn, is related to fewer depressive symptoms. (Lambert, Fincham, & Stillman, 2012)

Ready. Aim. Write.

#immaG

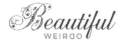

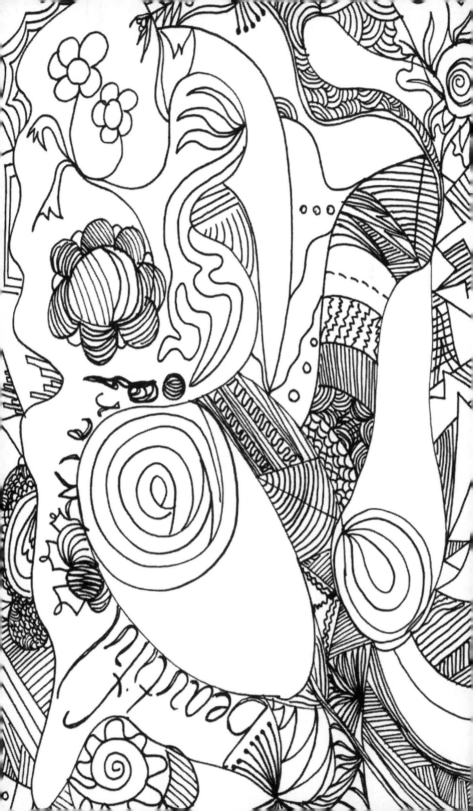

"GRATEFULNESS

IS THE KEY TO

LIVE A

SATISFYING

LIFE."

-T.C. Mason

I'm an innovative thinker as
I think outside of the box.

WHAT ARE YOU GRATEFUL FOR TODAY?

○ _____
○ _____
○ _____
○ _____

YEAH! I DID THAT!

I'm connecting with people wherever I go.
I'm humanity.

WHAT ARE YOU GRATEFUL FOR TODAY?

○ _____
○ _____
○ _____
○ _____

YEAH! I DID THAT!

I'm wise using my strengths &
delegating or outsourcing the rest.

○ _____

○ _____

○ _____

○ _____

YEAH! I DID THAT!

WHAT ARE YOU
GRATEFUL FOR TODAY?

I'm always blossoming &
I bear fresh fruit every month.

○ _____

○ _____

○ _____

○ _____

YEAH! I DID THAT!

WHAT ARE YOU
GRATEFUL FOR TODAY?

"WHEN WE FOCUS ON OUR GRATITUDE, THE TIDE OF DISAPPOINTMENT GOES OUT, AND THE TIDE OF LOVE RUSHES IN."

-Kirstin Armstrong

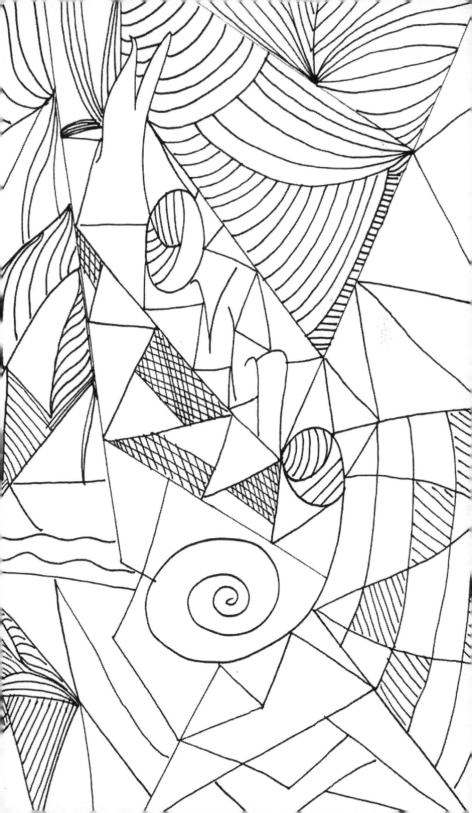

DATE

I'm remembering God's purpose & plan for my life no matter what obstacles come my way.

WHAT ARE YOU GRATEFUL FOR TODAY?

○ _____

○ _____

○ _____

○ _____

YEAH! I DID THAT!

DATE

I'm great because I am a creation of God.

WHAT ARE YOU GRATEFUL FOR TODAY?

○ _____

○ _____

○ _____

○ _____

YEAH! I DID THAT!

I'm discerning of marked moments & divine opportunities in my life.

- ○ _____
- ○ _____
- ○ _____
- ○ _____

YEAH! I DID THAT!

I'm sensitive to Holy Spirit & I'm in the right place at the right time.

- ○ _____
- ○ _____
- ○ _____
- ○ _____

YEAH! I DID THAT!

"NONE IS MORE
IMPOVERISHED THAN
THE ONE WHO HAS NO
GRATITUDE. GRATITUDE
IS A CURRENCY THAT
WE CAN ...
WITHOUT FEAR OF
BANKRUPTCY."

-Fred De Witt Van Amburgh

DID YOU KNOW...

Gratitude positively impacts an individual's overall well-being and connectedness.

There's a direct relationship between weekly benefit listing (i.e. writing down why you're grateful) and more positive optimism in life, an increase in exercising, less physical symptoms or ailments, high levels of positive affect, reports of pro-social behavior, more sleep, better sleep, and a sense of connectedness with others (Emmons &McCullough, 2003).

Ready. Aim. Write.

#immaG

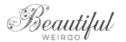

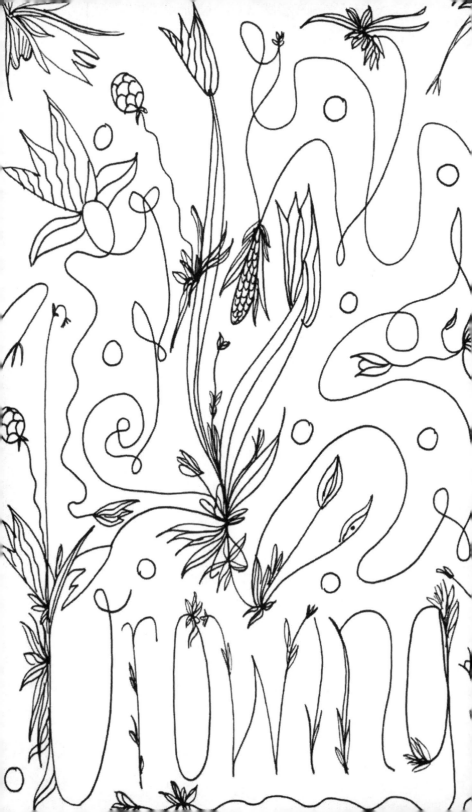

"WHEN I STARTED
COUNTING MY
BLESSINGS, MY
WHOLE LIFE TURNED
AROUND."

-Willie Nelson

DATE

I consistently speak words of life.

WHAT ARE YOU GRATEFUL FOR TODAY?

○ _____

○ _____

○ _____

○ _____

YEAH! I DID THAT!

DATE

I'm hearing God's voice in my decision making.

WHAT ARE YOU GRATEFUL FOR TODAY?

○ _____

○ _____

○ _____

○ _____

YEAH! I DID THAT!

I'm whole, nothing's missing & nothing's broken.

○ _____

○ _____

○ _____

○ _____

YEAH! I DID THAT!

I'm favored in every situation & I expect to receive random acts of kindness towards me.

○ _____

○ _____

○ _____

○ _____

YEAH! I DID THAT!

"BE THANKFUL FOR WHAT YOU HAVE; YOU'LL END UP HAVING MORE. IF YOU CONCENTRATE ON WHAT YOU DON'T HAVE, YOU WILL NEVER, EVER HAVE ENOUGH."

-Oprah Winfrey

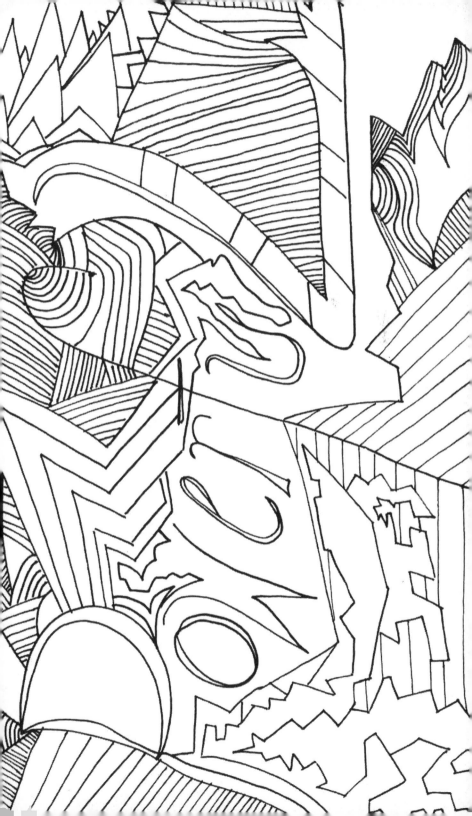

I'm embracing every day as a new opportunity to conquer life & make better decisions.

WHAT ARE YOU GRATEFUL FOR TODAY?

- ○ _____
- ○ _____
- ○ _____
- ○ _____

YEAH! I DID THAT!

I'm learning instruction from every experience & I'm implementing what I've learned.

WHAT ARE YOU GRATEFUL FOR TODAY?

- ○ _____
- ○ _____
- ○ _____
- ○ _____

YEAH! I DID THAT!

I'm accepting of where I am & where I'm going.

- ○ _____
- ○ _____
- ○ _____
- ○ _____

WHAT ARE YOU GRATEFUL FOR TODAY?

YEAH! I DID THAT!

I'm compassionate & extend myself to those in need.

- ○ _____
- ○ _____
- ○ _____
- ○ _____

WHAT ARE YOU GRATEFUL FOR TODAY?

YEAH! I DID THAT!

"HAPPINESS CANNOT BE TRAVELED TO, OWNED, EARNED, WORN OR CONSUMED. HAPPINESS IS THE SPIRITUAL EXPERIENCE OF LIVING EVERY MINUTE WITH LOVE, GRACE, AND GRATITUDE."

-Denis Waitley

DID YOU KNOW...

Gratitude is associated with "living the good life."

"Gratitude appears to potentially build feelings of subjective well-being and broaden the view of the good life" (p. 5). Gratitude appears to decrease materialism (Lambert, Fincham, Stillman, & Dean, 2009).

Ready. Aim. Write.

#immaG

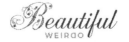

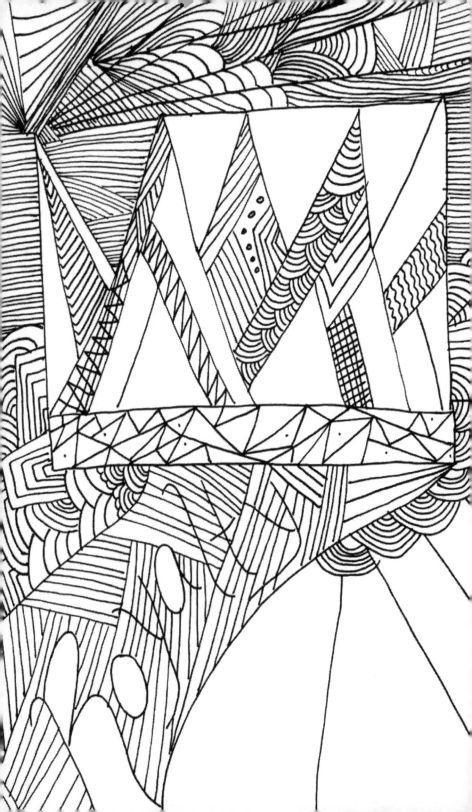

"IT'S NOT HAPPINESS
THAT BRINGS US
GRATITUDE. IT'S
GRATITUDE
THAT BRINGS US
HAPPINESS."

-Anonymous

I'm a work of art whose value is priceless.

WHAT ARE YOU GRATEFUL FOR TODAY?

- ◯ _____
- ◯ _____
- ◯ _____
- ◯ _____

YEAH! I DID THAT!

I'm humble & I ask for help when I need it.

WHAT ARE YOU GRATEFUL FOR TODAY?

- ◯ _____
- ◯ _____
- ◯ _____
- ◯ _____

YEAH! I DID THAT!

I'm saying "No" often, as it's a part of my self-care.

- ○ _____
- ○ _____
- ○ _____
- ○ _____

WHAT ARE YOU GRATEFUL FOR TODAY?

YEAH! I DID THAT!

I'm friendly & I attract people who appreciate my light.

- ○ _____
- ○ _____
- ○ _____
- ○ _____

WHAT ARE YOU GRATEFUL FOR TODAY?

YEAH! I DID THAT!

"GRATITUDE OPENS THE DOOR TO THE POWER, THE WISDOM, THE CREATIVITY OF THE UNIVERSE. YOU OPEN THE DOOR THROUGH GRATITUDE."

-Deepak Chopra

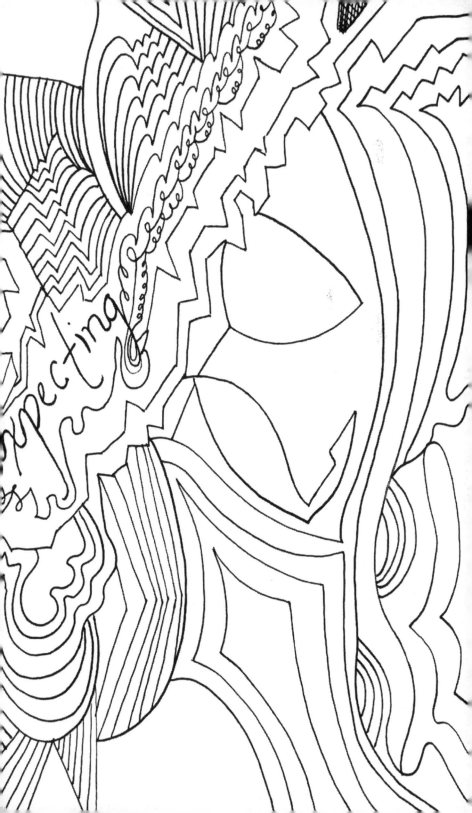

I'm inspecting the fruit in my life, keeping the good and addressing the bad.

WHAT ARE YOU GRATEFUL FOR TODAY?

- ○ _____
- ○ _____
- ○ _____
- ○ _____

YEAH! I DID THAT!

I consider & reconsider my actions to get to the truth of the matter as everything isn't always the way it seems.

WHAT ARE YOU GRATEFUL FOR TODAY?

- ○ _____
- ○ _____
- ○ _____
- ○ _____

YEAH! I DID THAT!

I'm mindfully shedding the weight of my past.

○ _____
○ _____
○ _____
○ _____

YEAH! I DID THAT!

WHAT ARE YOU GRATEFUL FOR TODAY?

I'm driving my life forward.

○ _____
○ _____
○ _____
○ _____

YEAH! I DID THAT!

WHAT ARE YOU GRATEFUL FOR TODAY?

Copyright © 2019 Beautiful Weirdo

"IT IS NOT JOY THAT
MAKES US GRATEFUL;
IT IS GRATITUDE THAT
MAKES US
JOYFUL."

- David Steindl-Rast

DID YOU KNOW...

Overall, general gratitude, is connected to better psychological functioning.

The benefits of being grateful are not limited to religious commitment (Rosmarin, Pirutinksy, Cohen, Galler, & Krumei, (2011).

Ready. Aim. Write.

#immaG

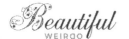

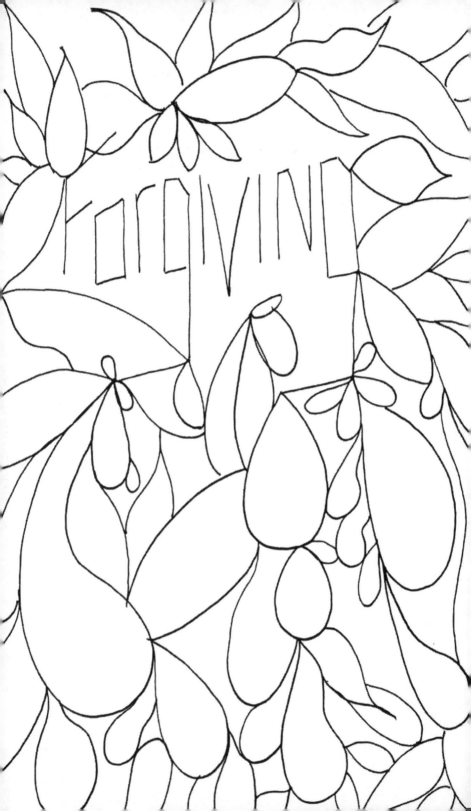

"IF YOU WANT TO FIND HAPPINESS, FIND GRATITUDE."

-Steve Maraboli

I'm focused & yet flexible enough to adapt to changes.

WHAT ARE YOU GRATEFUL FOR TODAY?

- ◯ _____
- ◯ _____
- ◯ _____
- ◯ _____

YEAH! I DID THAT!

I'm thriving & living a life of abundance & overflow in every area of my life.

WHAT ARE YOU GRATEFUL FOR TODAY?

- ◯ _____
- ◯ _____
- ◯ _____
- ◯ _____

YEAH! I DID THAT!

I'm thinking love & so I attract compassion.

○ _____
○ _____
○ _____
○ _____

WHAT ARE YOU GRATEFUL FOR TODAY?

YEAH! I DID THAT!

I'm intentionally creating spaces of joy, peace, & happiness.

○ _____
○ _____
○ _____
○ _____

WHAT ARE YOU GRATEFUL FOR TODAY?

YEAH! I DID THAT!

"FIND THE GOOD AND PRAISE IT."

-Alex Haley

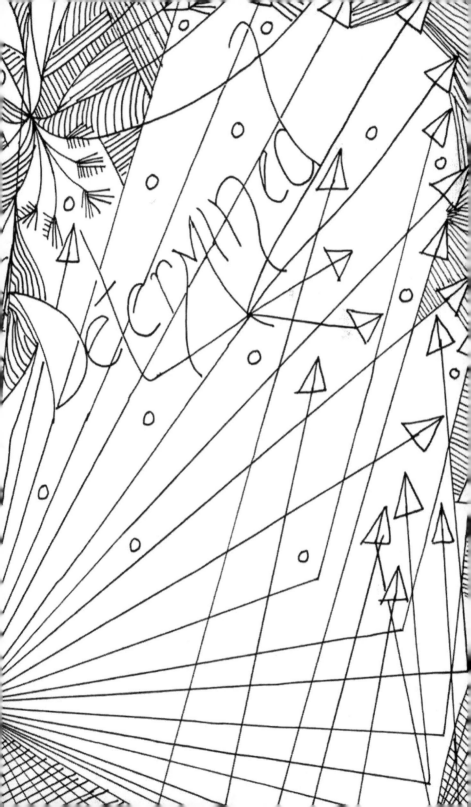

I'm rich in health, wealth, & wisdom.

WHAT ARE YOU GRATEFUL FOR TODAY?

- ◯ _____
- ◯ _____
- ◯ _____
- ◯ _____

YEAH! I DID THAT!

I'm seeing with eyes of faith & possibility in all situations.

WHAT ARE YOU GRATEFUL FOR TODAY?

- ◯ _____
- ◯ _____
- ◯ _____
- ◯ _____

YEAH! I DID THAT!

I'm aware of the intervals & changes in my life & so, I know when to walk, rest, & sprint.

- ◯ _____
- ◯ _____
- ◯ _____
- ◯ _____

YEAH! I DID THAT!

I'm disciplined & I'm going the distance. I'm forever challenging myself to do better than yesterday.

- ◯ _____
- ◯ _____
- ◯ _____
- ◯ _____

YEAH! I DID THAT!

"GRATITUDE CHANGES EVERYTHING."

-Anonymous

DID YOU KNOW...

Gratitude leads to a happier life.

Grateful individuals have at least three characteristics: sense of abundance, appreciation of simple pleasures, and an appreciation of other's contributions to one's well-being. Also, grateful individuals report being happier, having better moods, and positive affect (Watkins, Woodard, Stone, & Kolts, (2003).

Ready. Aim. Write.

#immaG

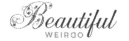

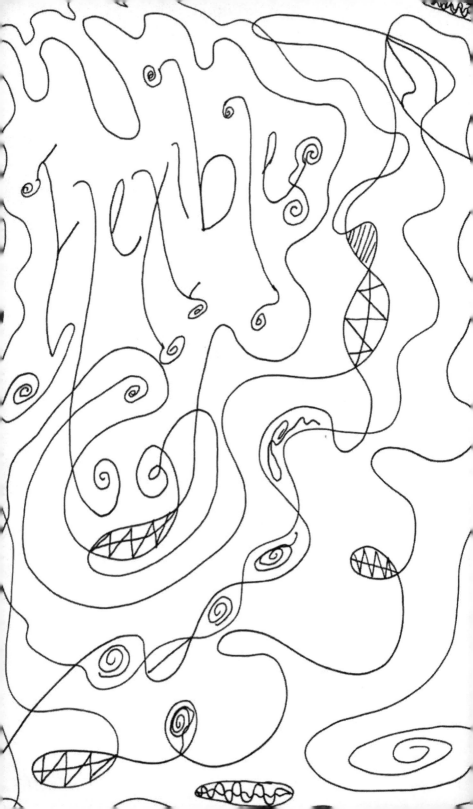

"MAY YOU WAKE WITH GRATITUDE."

-Anonymous

DATE

Through God, I'm building a legacy to change future generations.

WHAT ARE YOU GRATEFUL FOR TODAY?

○ _____

○ _____

○ _____

○ _____

YEAH! I DID THAT!

DATE

I'm rooted in love.

WHAT ARE YOU GRATEFUL FOR TODAY?

○ _____

○ _____

○ _____

○ _____

YEAH! I DID THAT!

I'm embracing & looking forward to the change in seasons in my life, both literally & figuratively!

○ _____
○ _____
○ _____
○ _____

YEAH! I DID THAT!

I'm greater than any challenging situations because God resides in me.

○ _____
○ _____
○ _____
○ _____

YEAH! I DID THAT!

"MY DAY BEGINS
AND ENDS WITH
GRATITUDE."

-Louise Hay

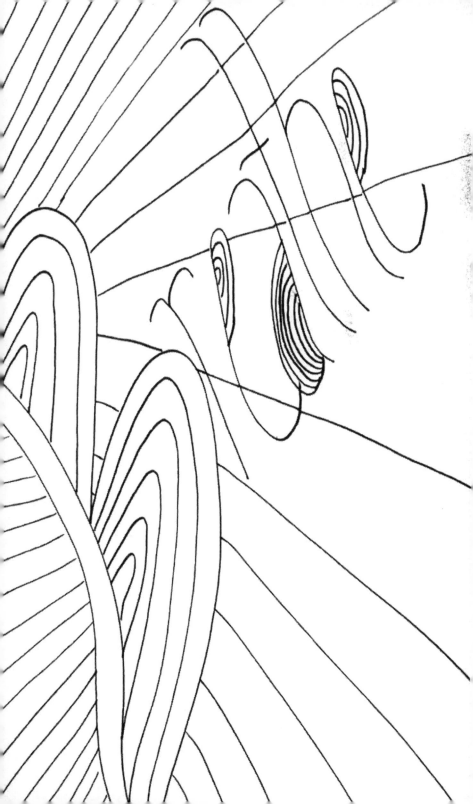

I'm a physical representation of love.

WHAT ARE YOU GRATEFUL FOR TODAY?

○ _____

○ _____

○ _____

○ _____

YEAH! I DID THAT!

I'm openly communicating even when I'm hurt. Vulnerability is my superpower.

WHAT ARE YOU GRATEFUL FOR TODAY?

○ _____

○ _____

○ _____

○ _____

YEAH! I DID THAT!

I'm using my gifts & talents to make the world better.

○ _____

○ _____

○ _____

○ _____

YEAH! I DID THAT!

I'm enjoying life and this moment in time.

○ _____

○ _____

○ _____

○ _____

YEAH! I DID THAT!

"THE ESSENCE OF ALL
BEAUTIFUL ART IS
GRATITUDE."

-Friedrich Nietzsche

DID YOU KNOW...

Gratitude leads to an increase in motivation to help others.

When helpers are thanked for their efforts the resulting sense of being socially valued are critical in encouraging them to provide more help in the future
(Grant & Gino, 2010).

Ready. Aim. Write.

#immaG

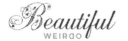

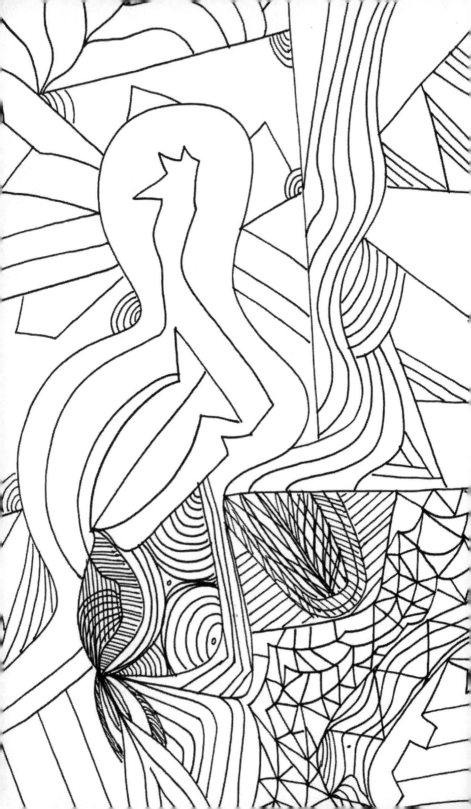

"THE MORE GRATEFUL
I AM, THE MORE
BEAUTY I SEE."

-Mary Davis

I quickly forgive those who have hurt me.

WHAT ARE YOU GRATEFUL FOR TODAY?

- ◯ _____
- ◯ _____
- ◯ _____
- ◯ _____

YEAH! I DID THAT!

I'm spending my life doing what I'm gifted to do.

WHAT ARE YOU GRATEFUL FOR TODAY?

- ◯ _____
- ◯ _____
- ◯ _____
- ◯ _____

YEAH! I DID THAT!

I'm the beauty God created.

○ _____
○ _____
○ _____
○ _____

YEAH! I DID THAT!

I'm living a life of joy, happiness, & confidence.

○ _____
○ _____
○ _____
○ _____

YEAH! I DID THAT!

GRATITUDE MAKES
SENSE OF YOUR PAST,
BRINGS PEACE
FOR TODAY, AND
CREATES A VISION FOR
TOMORROW.

-Melody Beattie

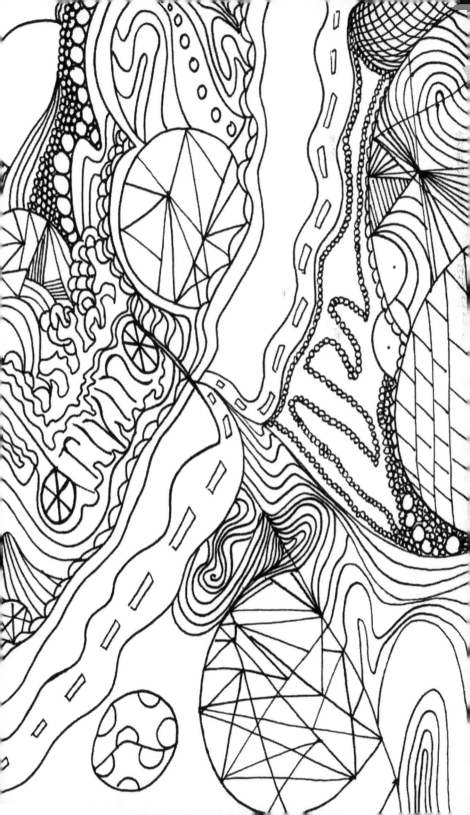

I'm sowing into the visions & dreams of people.

WHAT ARE YOU GRATEFUL FOR TODAY?

- ○ _____
- ○ _____
- ○ _____
- ○ _____

YEAH! I DID THAT!

I'm consistent in doing what will produce the best results in the end.

WHAT ARE YOU GRATEFUL FOR TODAY?

- ○ _____
- ○ _____
- ○ _____
- ○ _____

YEAH! I DID THAT!

I'm choosing behaviors that align with my expectations.

○ _____

○ _____

○ _____

○ _____

YEAH! I DID THAT!

WHAT ARE YOU GRATEFUL FOR TODAY?

I'm planning prosperity & success in every area of my life.

○ _____

○ _____

○ _____

○ _____

YEAH! I DID THAT!

WHAT ARE YOU GRATEFUL FOR TODAY?

"THERE ARE ALWAYS FLOWERS FOR THOSE WHO WANT TO SEE THEM."

-Henri Matisse

DID YOU KNOW...

Gratitude increases positive emotions.

Gratefulness helps build social connectedness and presence of meaning in life, which in effect increases subjective well-being (Liao, 2018).

Ready. Aim. Write.

#immaG

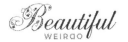

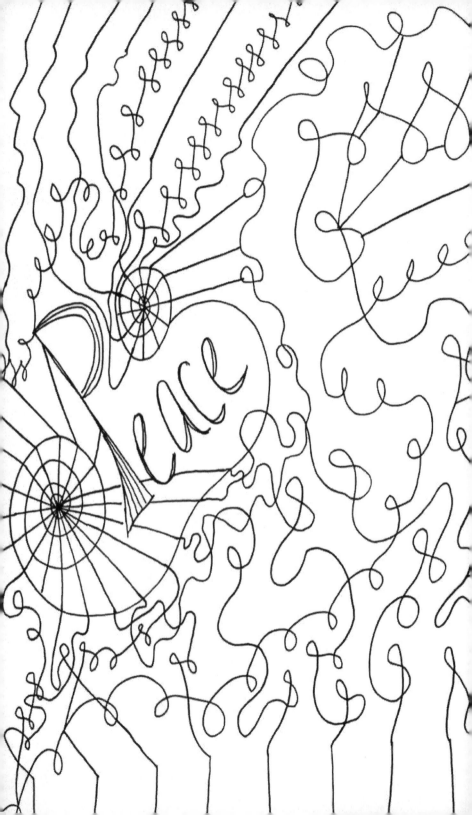

"GRATITUDE CAN
TRANSFORM
COMMON DAYS INTO
THANKSGIVINGS, TURN
ROUTINE JOBS INTO JOY,
AND CHANGE ORDINARY
OPPORTUNITIES INTO
BLESSINGS."

-William Arthur Ward

I'm learning to become better at being me every day.

WHAT ARE YOU GRATEFUL FOR TODAY?

- ○ _____
- ○ _____
- ○ _____
- ○ _____

YEAH! I DID THAT!

I'm partnered with people who want to see me grow & succeed.

WHAT ARE YOU GRATEFUL FOR TODAY?

- ○ _____
- ○ _____
- ○ _____
- ○ _____

YEAH! I DID THAT!

I'm bringing joy to myself & joy to those around me.

○ _____

○ _____

○ _____

○ _____

YEAH! I DID THAT!

WHAT ARE YOU
GRATEFUL FOR TODAY?

*I'm accepting that I don't
have to be right all the time.*

○ _____

○ _____

○ _____

○ _____

YEAH! I DID THAT!

WHAT ARE YOU
GRATEFUL FOR TODAY?

"WEAR GRATITUDE LIKE A CLOAK, AND IT WILL FEED EVERY CORNER OF YOUR LIFE."

-Rumi

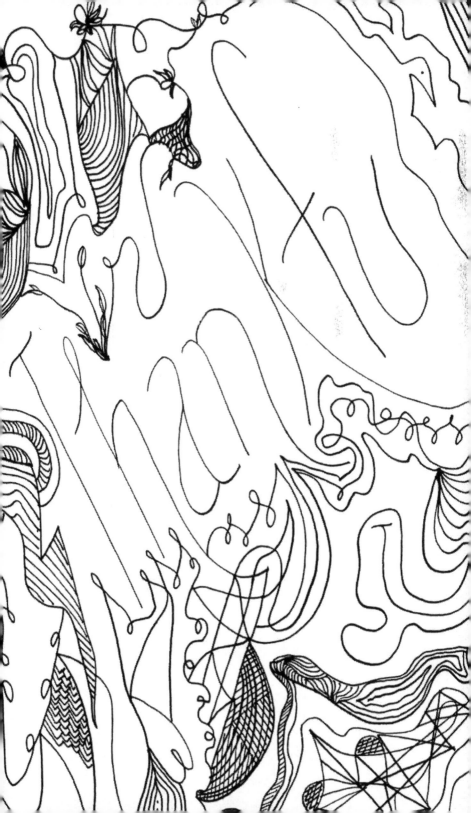

I'm everything that I dreamed & hope I'd be & this is just the beginning. I'm a manifestation of faith & God's word.

WHAT ARE YOU GRATEFUL FOR TODAY?

- ○ _____
- ○ _____
- ○ _____
- ○ _____

YEAH! I DID THAT!

I'm faithful on average days.
I'm faithful on extraordinary days.

WHAT ARE YOU GRATEFUL FOR TODAY?

- ○ _____
- ○ _____
- ○ _____
- ○ _____

YEAH! I DID THAT!

I'm loved & my entire body vibrates
& exudes love. I'm contagious.

○ _____
○ _____
○ _____
○ _____

YEAH! I DID THAT!

WHAT ARE YOU
GRATEFUL FOR TODAY?

I'm honest with myself &
so I'm honest with others.

○ _____
○ _____
○ _____
○ _____

YEAH! I DID THAT!

WHAT ARE YOU
GRATEFUL FOR TODAY?

"SHOWING GRATITUDE
IS ONE OF THE
SIMPLEST YET MOST
POWERFUL THINGS
HUMANS CAN DO FOR
EACH OTHER."

-Randy Rausch

DID YOU KNOW...

Gratitude reduces depressive symptoms

Gratitude decreases reports of depressive symptoms by prompting people to reframe otherwise negative experiences as potentially positive experiences. This reframing, in turn, is related to fewer depressive symptoms. (Lambert, Fincham, & Stillman, 2012)

Ready. Aim. Write

#immaG

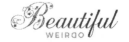

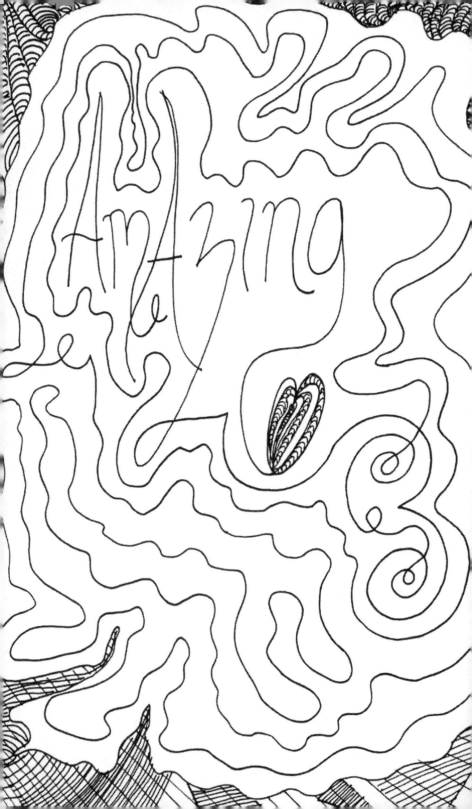

"NO MATTER WHAT
THE SITUATION IS...
CLOSE YOUR EYES
AND THINK OF ALL
OF THE THINGS IN
YOUR LIFE YOU
COULD BE GRATEFUL
FOR RIGHT NOW."

-Deepak Chopra

I'm a listener & follower of Holy Spirit.

WHAT ARE YOU GRATEFUL FOR TODAY?

- ○ _____
- ○ _____
- ○ _____
- ○ _____

YEAH! I DID THAT!

My mouth is powerful & it produces life, so I guard the words that come out of it.

WHAT ARE YOU GRATEFUL FOR TODAY?

- ○ _____
- ○ _____
- ○ _____
- ○ _____

YEAH! I DID THAT!

I'm greater than my past.

○ _____

○ _____

○ _____

○ _____

YEAH! I DID THAT!

I'm my wildest dreams and attract a tribe who support me.

○ _____

○ _____

○ _____

○ _____

YEAH! I DID THAT!

"START EACH DAY
WITH A POSITIVE
THOUGHT AND A
GRATEFUL HEART."

-Roy T. Bennett

DID YOU KNOW...

Gratitude reduces depressive symptoms

"When falling asleep, grateful people are less likely
to think negative and worrying thoughts,
and more likely to think positive thoughts
(Wood, Joseph, Lloyd, & Atkins, 2009, p. 46)."

Ready. Aim. Write.

#immaG

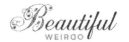

I'm authentic and true to myself.

WHAT ARE YOU GRATEFUL FOR TODAY?

○ _____

○ _____

○ _____

○ _____

YEAH! I DID THAT!

I'm living my life & nobody else's.

WHAT ARE YOU GRATEFUL FOR TODAY?

○ _____

○ _____

○ _____

○ _____

YEAH! I DID THAT!

I'm kind to myself as I take the time to heal.

○ _____

○ _____

○ _____

○ _____

WHAT ARE YOU GRATEFUL FOR TODAY?

YEAH! I DID THAT!

I'm precious & worthy to be protected.

○ _____

○ _____

○ _____

○ _____

WHAT ARE YOU GRATEFUL FOR TODAY?

YEAH! I DID THAT!

"THIS IS A
WONDERFUL DAY.
I'VE NEVER SEEN
THIS ONE BEFORE."

-Maya Angelou

DID YOU KNOW...

**Gratitude reduces negative affect
(i.e. negative emotions)**

Focusing on one's blessings and being grateful leads
to a reduction in negative emotions

(Emmons & McCullough, 2003)

Ready. Aim. Write.

#immaG

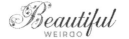

I'm mature enough to trust God even when things aren't going my way.

WHAT ARE YOU GRATEFUL FOR TODAY?

- ○ _____
- ○ _____
- ○ _____
- ○ _____

YEAH! I DID THAT!

I'm creating the life I want to live.

WHAT ARE YOU GRATEFUL FOR TODAY?

- ○ _____
- ○ _____
- ○ _____
- ○ _____

YEAH! I DID THAT!

I'm forgiving myself for being unforgiving in areas of my life.

DATE

○ _____
○ _____
○ _____
○ _____

YEAH! I DID THAT!

WHAT ARE YOU GRATEFUL FOR TODAY?

I'm seeing with eyes of faith like never before.

DATE

○ _____
○ _____
○ _____
○ _____

YEAH! I DID THAT!

WHAT ARE YOU GRATEFUL FOR TODAY?

Copyright © 2019 Beautiful Weirdo

DATE

I'm praying & giving thanks in everything.

WHAT ARE YOU GRATEFUL FOR TODAY?

- ○ _____
- ○ _____
- ○ _____
- ○ _____

YEAH! I DID THAT!

DATE

I'm steadily clipping the dead ends from my life. I'm growing.

WHAT ARE YOU GRATEFUL FOR TODAY?

- ○ _____
- ○ _____
- ○ _____
- ○ _____

YEAH! I DID THAT!

"GRATITUDE FOR THE PRESENT MOMENT AND THE FULLNESS OF LIFE NOW IS TRUE PROSPERITY."

-Eckhart Tolle

YOU DID THAT!!

Congratulations! You have just finished 3 months of gratitude! What did you learn? Did you notice any changes? YOU ARE INCREDIBLE, and I am so grateful that you stuck with this process. You invested in yourself!! **YOU DID THAT & IT'S TIME TO CELEBRATE!**

I ask one small favor of you, please email tcmason@ imabeautifulweirdo.com and tell me about your experience. Feel free to send along a photo of how you celebrated #immaG!

Thank-you for taking the time to **READY. AIM. WRITE.** and use the power of gratitude as a weapon in this war on stressors and depression. Never be caught unarmed! Keep it Up!

Bring the *Armed With Gratefulness* Gratitude workshop to your area

tcmason@imabeautifulweirdo.com

Follow on Social Media

Facebook: imabeautifulweirdo

Instagram: @imabeautifulweirdo

#beautifulweirdo #immaG

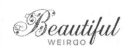

GRATEFULNESS REFERENCES

Emmons, R. A., & McCullough, M. E. (2003). Counting blessings versus burdens: An experimental investigation of gratitude and subjective well-being in daily life. Journal of Personality and Social Psychology, 84(2), 377-389. doi: 10.1111/j.1467-6494.2004.00305.x

Grant, A. M., & Gino, F. (2010). A little thanks goes a long way: Explaining why gratitude expressions motivate prosocial behavior. Journal of Personality and Social Psychology, 98(6), 946-9. doi: http://dx.doi.org.library.capella.edu/10.1037/a0017935

Lambert, N. M., Fincham, F.D., & Stillman, T.F. (2012). Gratitude and depressive symptoms: The role of positive reframing and positive emotion. Cognition and Emotion, 26(4), 615-633. doi: 10.1080/02699931.2011.595393

Lambert, N. M., Fincham, F. D., Stillman, T. F., & Dean, L. R. (2009). More gratitude, less materialism: The mediating role of life satisfaction. The Journal of Positive Psychology, 4(1), 32-42. doi: 10.1080/17439760802216311

Liao, K. Y. (2018). Gratefulness and subjective well-being: Social connectedness and presence of meaning as mediators. Journal of Counseling Psychology,65(3), 383-393. doi: http://dx.doi.org.library.capella.edu/10.1037/cou0000271

GRATEFULNESS REFERENCES

McCollough, M. E., Emmons, R. A., Tsang, J. (2002). The grateful disposition: A conceptual and empirical topography. Journal of Personality and Social Psychology, 82(1), 112-127. doi: http://dx.doi.org.library.capella.edu/10.1037/0022-3514.82.1.112

Murray, J.L., & Lopez, A.D. (1996). The global burden of disease: A comprehensive assessment of mortality and disability from diseases, injuries and risk factors in 1990 and projected to 2020. Retrieved from https://apps.who.int/iris/bitstreamhandle/10665/41864/0965546608_eng.pdf

Rosmarin, D. H., Pirutinksy, S., Cohen, A. B., Galler, Y., & Krumei, E. J. (2011). Grateful to God or just plain grateful? A comparison of religious and general gratitude. The Journal of Positive Psychology, 6(5), 389-396. doi: 10.1080/17439760.2011.596557

Southwick, S.M., Vythilingam, M., & Charney, D. S. (2005). The psychobiology of depression and resilience to stress: Implications for prevention and treatment. Annual Review of Clinical Psychology, 1, 255-291.

Watkins, P. C., Woodard, K., Stone, T., & Kolts, R. L. (2003). Gratitude and happiness: Development of a measure of gratitude, and relationships with subjective well-being. Social Behavior and Personality, 31(5), 431-451. doi: 10.2224/sbp.2003.31.5.431

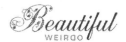